Contents

Foreword

We all want to see our dogs live a long, happy, disease-free life and diet is one of the most important factors in achieving this.

The 'Book of Home Pets' published in 1862, notes that 'not one of our catalogue of pets stands so likely a chance of being killed by kindness as the dog.' The same is true today.

The aim of this booklet is to look at the bewildering number of theories on diet, all assuring us that their way is right. It will provide information on the nutritional requirements of dogs and how they are obtained. We shall look at their provision in commercial foods and examine the pros and cons of raw and home-cooked foods so that you may make an informed decision on how best to provide a balanced diet for your dog in a manner that suits your budget and lifestyle.

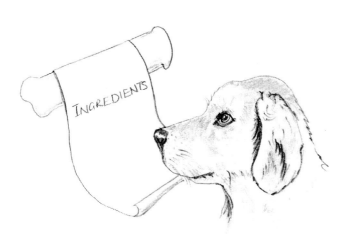

Why Diet is Important

There is more to food than just providing fuel. Although this is its primary function, the **type** of fuel we feed our dogs is the foundation of their health and will determine how they look, feel and behave; whether they will be nervous, tired, fearful or confident, happy and active.

Pleasant surroundings, good food and peace of mind favour digestion in your dog's body, allowing the optimum uptake of the available nutrients.

In broad terms there are four main causes of disease.

- **Lack of proper nutrients.**
  A malnourished body, and by this we mean a body that is not receiving the correct balance and quantities of nutrients, is less efficient in dealing with its waste products so that they gradually build up allowing disease causing bacteria to flourish leading to toxaemia and contamination.

- **Toxaemia and contamination of the body.**

  Where there is a strong and healthy immune system it is much more difficult for pathogenic viruses and disease carrying organisms to gain a stronghold

- **Hereditary disease.**

  Hereditary conditions, whilst impossible to eliminate can be managed and improved with good nutrition. Allergies and diabetes are two such conditions that can benefit from a balanced diet.

- **Negative state of mind.**

  Negative states of mind can be helped by diet as well as by environment and a loving bond between dog and owner. Specific vitamins, minerals and amino acids are necessary for the brain to send messages to nerve cells and thus influence the general feeling of well being which in turn affects behaviour.

Most common diseases are caused by the deficiencies of nutrients in the body that develop gradually over years of eating a imbalanced diet. Therefore, if we feed our dogs a balanced diet we can help them enjoy life to the full and live to a ripe old age.

The digestive system is very complex and may be subject to many physical and chemical abnormalities. It is imperative that expert advice should be sought from your Vet in any case of abnormal situation or alteration to the dogs' normal eating habits.

What your dog needs

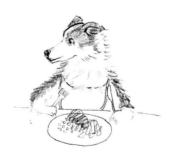

The basic building blocks of a healthy diet are water, protein, fats, carbohydrates and the micronutrients – vitamins, and minerals; all these are needed in the correct proportions to ensure optimum health.

Water

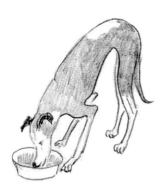

Water is essential to life and is part of every function of the body. Fresh, good quality water should be available at all times as it is necessary for digestive, absorptive, circulatory, and excretory functions. It transports nutrients including water soluble vitamins into the body's cells and waste matter out.

The taste of tap water is not always to our dogs' liking and they sometimes prefer to drink rainwater. This is fine as long as the rainwater is bacteria free. The taste of tap water varies from area to area and, if you are concerned, can be improved either by filtering or by keeping it in a jug for a short time to allow the taste and smell of the various chemicals that water companies love to add to dissipate. The chemical content of the water will be the same but it will taste better. When walking in the countryside dogs will often drink from rivers, streams or puddles so be sure that such sources are clean and unpolluted. Water that runs through sheep grazing is to be avoided as there is a substantial risk of fluke worm. Therefore it is important, when doing a country or seaside walk, to carry water for your dog rather than hope to find some en route.

Protein

Proteins are the building blocks, not just of tissues, but also of hormones, enzymes and blood formation. They also serve as a source of heat and energy.

Proteins are very complex; they are made up of various combinations of 24 amino acids, eight of which are essential for life. During digestion proteins present in foods break down into amino acids that maintain, repair and replace cells throughout the body. Foods that contain the eight essential amino acids are known as complete proteins and are found in meat, fish eggs and dairy products. If no complete proteins are fed care must be taken to ensure that the eight essential amino acids are fed in each meal, but unless you are trying to make your dog a vegetarian this is unlikely to be a problem.

Puppies need a greater percentage of protein in their diet as they are essential for growth, but the adult dog also needs adequate protein intake for repairs and renewals of everyday wear and tear and to give the energy required to maintain the daily activities.

The symptoms of protein deficiency are many and varied. Poor growth rate in puppies, poor coat, susceptibility to infection, fatigue, depression and slow healing of wounds, all indicate an inadequate amount of protein in a dog's diet. In adult dogs protein deficiency can lead to faulty cell function and a lack of iron and calcium may develop causing problems ranging from tooth decay to premature aging and cancer.

Excessive protein consumption can be just as problematical to health as too little. It can lead to kidney problems, heart disease, and arthritis. Behaviour problems can also arise when the dog is fed too much protein in relation to the amount of energy it expends. If we provide a lot of energy but no out let for it then we can see over excited and hyper-active dogs.

Fats

Despite their reputation as a cause of obesity and a source of cholesterol, fats play a vital role in bodily functions. Fats help the system to absorb and transport vitamins A, D, E, K and the mineral Calcium. Certain types insulate the nerves, ensuring a healthy flow of nerve impulses without which irritability and nervous disorders occur. All cell membranes contain fats and, most importantly fats are needed to form the hormones, which are essential to a vast range of bodily functions.

Fats are broken down by digestion into glycerol and fatty acids. The body can manufacture most of these acids. The exceptions are three which are known as essential fatty acids and **must** be supplied by the food we feed our dogs. There are two basic categories of Essential Fatty Acids – Omega 3 and Omega 6. Omega 3 is found in salmon, herring, sardines, mackerel and flax seeds or oil. Omega 6 is found in nuts seeds, legumes and in unsaturated vegetable oils.

There are three major categories of fatty acids; saturated, polyunsaturated and monounsaturated. Saturated fatty acids are found mostly in animal products such as meat and dairy products and also in coconut oil and vegetable shortening (dogs are unlikely to find either of the last two palatable). Polyunsaturated fatty acids are found in corn, soya, safflower and sunflower oils and also in certain fish oils. Monounsaturated fatty acids are found mostly in vegetable and nut oils such as olive and peanut oil.

The more unsaturated the fat, the easier it is for the body to process and use it rather than stockpile it as body fat. It would be wrong to think that saturated fats should be totally avoided. The important thing is to balance them with polyunsaturated oils.

Rancid oil is to be avoided. It is important to store oil in an airtight bottle away from light as the oxidisation process converts unsaturated fats into saturated fatty acids. **Rancid oils are toxic,** not only in their own right, but also when contained in grains, legumes, nuts and seeds. Recent studies have found that rancid oils deactivate vitamin E and can cause toxic substances that damage to the digestive tract, in some cases causing ulcers and contributing to premature ageing, arthritis, heart problems and cancer.

Your dog needs *some* fat in his diet. Most sources recommend a daily intake of between ¼ ounce for maintenance and ½ ounce for moderate work in a 33-lb/15 kg dog. Your dog will understandably find animal fat more palatable, but care must be taken to include essential fatty acids in the diet. Anti oxidants such as vitamin E should be fed to dogs that have a high intake of polyunsaturated fats. If fed in excess these fats can go rancid in the body. Lecithin containing foods improve the digestion of fats.

Cholesterol is not as much a problem for dogs as it is for humans as their systems have the ability to deal with excessive amounts and eliminate them from the body. It has been discovered that dogs only develop atherosclerotic lesions where their thyroid function is depressed. However if too much saturated fat is given it will be stored as body fat.

Do not feed your dog margarine as the hydrogenisation process changes fatty acids to a form foreign to most mammals. There is good evidence to suggest that extensive use of such products contribute to an increased risk of ill health.

Carbohydrates

Carbohydrates are an essential macronutrient. They supply the body with energy and are the main source of blood glucose, a major supplier of energy and stimulator of healthy red blood cell production. A major fuel for other cell functions, they are plentiful in plants fruits grains and legumes, honey and sugar.

There are two groups of carbohydrates; simple and complex. Simple carbohydrates, the fast energy releasers, sometimes known as simple sugars are found in fruit – fructose or fruit sugars, milk – lactose or milk sugars and table sugar – sucrose. Complex carbohydrates are also sugars but have longer chains of molecules and are gradually broken down by the body into simple sugars, which gives a slower release of energy over a much longer period, and this helps with blood sugar control.

Carbohydrate intake should always be in the form of unrefined foods – these are natural unprocessed fruits, vegetables, peas, beans and whole grain products. These foods have the advantage over refined foods in that they contain a wide range of other nutrients that help in the utilisation of the sugars. Problems with carbohydrates begin when they are refined and stripped of most of their vitamin and mineral content leaving them with little food value. If eaten in excess they can lead to a number of disorders such as diabetes, hypoglycaemia and candida infections. Unrefined carbohydrates of course retain that very important feature dietary fibre or what used to be known as roughage. Most fibre is not digested but is water-soluble. As it passes through the digestive tract it acts as a cleaner gathering up the substances that result in the production of cholesterol. It also helps produce bulkier stools, which prevent constipation.

In the wild, dogs obtain the carbohydrate in their diet from fruit and vegetables. They will eat ripe or over ripe fruit as it is easily digested. Rotten fruit is to be avoided because it can contain the botulism bacteria and cause paralysis. If your dog enjoys fruit this is a good source of simple sugars, fibre and various vitamins, minerals and enzymes. Under ripe fruits are difficult for a dog to digest as their digestive system has difficulty in breaking down the cell walls. Therefore if you want to feed fruits that are firm but not fully ripe the best way is to put them through a food processor or juicer. This crushes the cell wall allowing nutrients to be absorbed. Vegetables should be treated in the same way. The natural way for dogs to take in vegetable matter is to eat the semi-digested matter they find in the gut of their prey. That said, in the 10,000 years or more that dogs have been companions to man, part of their diet has been left overs. Their systems are adapting to grain and cooked vegetables but in the wild such items would be unrefined and constitute only a small part of their total food intake. It is our modern refined carbohydrates that are so bad for both our dogs and us.

Vitamins

Vitamins are found in small and varying amounts in all natural vegetable and animal foods. About 20 vitamins are known to be vital for healthy nutrition. They are functionally interrelated and work synergistically with each other and certain minerals to help detoxification and optimum organ function thereby playing an important role in energy release and promotion of longevity.

Most vitamins are water-soluble and any surplus can be eliminated by urination, but fat-soluble vitamins are harder to eliminate and accumulate by being stored in body fat so in the overweight dog it is wise to be aware that some adverse effects may be seen.

The level of vitamins needed by each individual is determined by age, sex, metabolic rate and the amount of work / exercise the dog is doing. This can vary tremendously from dog to dog; you may have two dogs that seem identical in terms of breed, age, sex and the amount of work, yet their individual requirements may be completely different.

Below is a list of major vitamins, what they do and where they are found and the recommended daily allowance for an adult dog weighing 33lbs / 15kg and consuming 1,000 calories a day.

g = grams; mg = milligrams; ug = micrograms

Vitamins A and E are usually measured in i.u.(international units) these are a measure of potency.

Vitamins

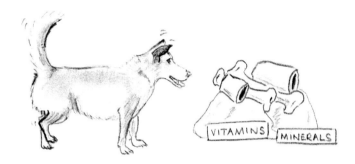

Vitamin A   RDA 379ug

Important for development and fertility. Needed for healthy skin and protection from infections. It is an antioxidant and immune system booster. It is essential for vision, especially night vision and also for trans membrane protein transfer.

Found in liver, carrots, watercress, cabbage, broccoli and tomatoes.

Vitamin B1 (Thiamin)   RDA 0.56mg

Essential for energy production, carbohydrate metabolism and nerve function. It can help prevent arthritis and arteriosclerosis and can be useful in overcoming stress and depression.

Found in brewer's yeast, whole grains, particularly brown rice, lamb, peas, lettuce, cabbage, cauliflower, beans and tomato

Vitamin B2 (Riboflavin)   RDA 1.3mg

Needed to repair and maintain healthy skin. Important for coat, claws and eyes. Helps with enzyme functions. Found in Watercress, cabbage, broccoli, mackerel, milk, liver, fish and eggs

Vitamin B3 (Niacin)   RDA 4mg

Essential for enzyme functions, helping to regulate blood sugar and cholesterol levels. It is essential for energy production, brain function and the skin. It is vital for a healthy nervous system.

Found in tuna, chicken, salmon, cabbage, lamb, mackerel, turkey, courgettes, sunflower seeds and wheatgerm

Vitamin B5 (Pantothenic Acid)   RDA 4mg

Involved in a number of metabolic functions and the production. Essential for brain and nerve function. Maintains healthy skin and fur.

Found in royal jelly, cod's roe, organ meats, wheatgerm, wholegrains, broccoli, cabbage, celery and eggs.

Vitamin B6   RDA 0.4mg

Involved with more than sixty enzymes it is essential for glucose generation, red blood cell function, niacin synthesis, nervous system function, immune response, hormone regulation and gene activation. It is a natural anti-depressant and diuretic.

Found in brewer's yeast, liver, kidney, sunflower seeds, wheatgerm, cauliflower, cabbage and eggs.

Vitamin B12   RDA 9ug

Essential for the functioning of all cells, mainly involved in energy metabolism, nerve function and immune function. It is responsible, with folic acid for the formation of red blood cells.

Found in liver, kidneys, sardines, eggs, tuna, cottage cheese, Spirulina and bee pollen

Folic Acid   RDA 68ug

Crucial to the production of red blood cells and for the proper cell division of DNA, it is essential during pregnancy for the development of brain and nerves of the foetus. It also stimulates stomach secretions improving digestion. It promotes mental and emotional health by helping the body to produce the chemicals that transmit messages between the nerve cells.

Found in wheat germ, brewer's yeast, spinach, kale, sprouts broccoli, peanuts, cashew nuts and egg yolks

Choline   RDA 425 mg

Helps break down fats and transports fats to the cells. It is needed for nerve transmission and liver function. It is vital for learning and memory.

Found in lecithin, eggs, fish, liver, whole grains, and leafy green vegetables.

Vitamin C No RDA

Dogs make their own vitamin C but research suggests that a good intake is beneficial as it strengthens the immune system. It is a powerful antioxidant, protecting against age related diseases from cancer to heart disease. It is an antihistamine, and as an antipollutant detoxifies the body.

Found in peppers, broccoli sprouts, cabbage, cauliflower, peas and tomatoes.

Vitamin D RDA 3. 4ug

Promotes the absorption of calcium and phosphorus, both of which are essential for strong and healthy bones. It also helps the assimilation of vitamin A and maintains a healthy nervous system, a regular heartbeat and efficient blood clotting.

Found in sunshine, fish liver oil, herrings, sardines, mackerel, salmon, cottage cheese and eggs

Vitamin E RDA 100 i.u.

An important antioxidant protects cells from damage. It improves cell respiration helping to prevent blood clots and thrombosis. It improves wound healing and fertility and is good for the skin.

Found in unrefined vegetable oils, sunflower seeds wheatgerm, tuna, salmon, whole grains and eggs.

Vitamin K   RDA 0.41mg

Activates blood clotting factors. Promotes healthy bones.

Found in kale cauliflower, sprouts, cabbage, lettuce, spinach, egg yolk and yoghurt.

Minerals

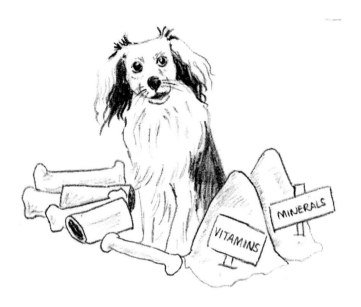

Minerals are elements found in the earth's crust and in a process taking millions of years, form the basis of soil from which they are absorbed by plants and then eaten by herbivorous animals. Thus we absorb minerals by eating vegetables or animals. Poor soil has a lack of minerals and if we eat foods grown on such ground our mineral levels will be depleted.

Minerals and trace elements are vital for good health and well being as they are involved in various enzyme systems which enable the proper digestion and absorption of foods enabling the body to perform its functions including energy production, brain function, growth and healing.

Calcium, phosphorus, potassium, sodium, magnesium and silicon are required in quite large quantities and are referred to as bulk minerals. Trace element minerals are, although required in very small amounts, vitally important for good health, they are Boron, Chromium, Copper, Germanium, Iodine, Iron, Sulphur and Zinc. Whilst these elements are indispensable to the body, excesses are undesirable.

The proper balance of minerals is important. The level of each mineral in the body has an effect on every other, so if one is out of balance all mineral levels are affected and if not corrected can lead to illness. It is important to feed a wide variety of foods to ensure that a good range of minerals is ingested as some compete with each other for absorption whist some work synchronistically with each other. If you are concerned that the food you are feeding has mineral deficiencies due to being produced on poor soil or by the refining process (this can remove up to 90% of the trace minerals) you may consider supplementing the diet. If this is the case it is important to give a good quality multi-mineral which aims to keep the required balance.

The following table lists the main minerals and the jobs they do.

The amounts shown are the daily requirements for an adult dog weighing 33lbs/15kgs

Consuming 1,000 calories a day

g = gms; mg = milligrams; ug = micrograms

Minerals

Calcium   RDA 0.75g

Normalizes nerve and muscle function, regulates heartbeat, improves blood clotting. Promotes skin, bone and teeth formation and maintains the correct acid-alkaline balance. Needs vitamins A, C and D, magnesium in the ration 3:2 and phosphorus in the ratio 2:1 for proper absorption. Exercise helps calcium deposition in the bones.

Found in dairy products, brewer's yeast, parsley, prunes, cabbage, sesame seeds and sunflower seeds.

Chromium   RDA 10mcg

Essential for the correct metabolism of glucose and cholesterol. It is the main constituent of the glucose tolerance factor which balances blood sugar and can help to normalise hunger. It helps protect DNA and RNA and is essential for heart function.

Found in brewer's yeast, wholemeal or rye flours, wheatgerm, eggs, chicken, apples parsnips and lamb.

Phosphorus   RDA 0.75g

Combines with calcium to form and maintain bone and teeth. It is a constituent of DNA and of myelin which insulates the nerves. It aids metabolism and energy production and helps maintain the acid-alkaline balance of the body.

Found in almost all foods.

Magnesium   RDA 150mg

Maintains strong bones and tooth enamel, promotes muscle and nerve cell membrane stability so is important for heart muscles and nervous system. Is essential for energy production and hormone secretion and function. It is an important factor in many enzyme functions.

Found in wheatgerm, brewer's yeast, buckwheat flour, nuts, peas, and apples.

Sodium   RDA100mg

Maintains osmotic pressure in tissues, preventing dehydration. Helps nerve functioning, used in muscle contraction, including the heart. Helps move nutrients and oxygen in and out of the cells. Keeps calcium soluble.

Found in miso, beetroot, celery, cabbage, cottage cheese, kelp, watercress, carrots and meat. There should be sufficient in most foods to meet the daily requirements, but care must be taken when feeding commercial or processed foods as their salt content is very high and excess sodium can be a cause of kidney damage.

Potassium   RDA 1g

Works with sodium to regulate water retention and stimulate the kidneys. It is involved in insulin secretion and nerve impulse transmission. Promotes waste elimination, enhances mental alertness, and reduces blood pressure.

Found in watercress, endive, cabbage, celery, parsley, courgettes, cauliflower, pumpkin, and bananas.

Iron   7.5mg

Indispensable for the production of haemoglobin, the red pigment in blood that transports oxygen and carbon dioxide to and from the cells. It is a component of several enzymes and is vital for energy production.

Found in liver, meat, oatmeal, brewer's yeast, pumpkin seeds, parsley.

Copper   RDA 1.5mg

Aids the absorption of iron. Helps connective tissue formation, melanin pigment formation, and myelin formation. It is involved in many enzyme activities. Small excesses can be a cause for concern as most water now is delivered by copper piping. Running the tap for a couple of minutes, especially in the mornings, or using filtered water overcomes this problem. Zinc helps reduce excess copper levels.

Found in whole wheat, liver, and molasses.

Zinc   RDA 15mg

Zinc is an essential trace element and a component of over 200 enzymes. It takes part in the metabolism of carbohydrates, proteins and the synthesis of DNA and RNA. It aids the ability to cope with stress, and combines with vitamins A, B6 and B12 to promote cell replication, so helping wound healing. It helps reduce excess copper and inhibits histamine production.

Found in meat, ginger root, haddock, brewer's yeast, pumpkin seeds, peas, turnips, egg yolk, wholewheat grain, rye, oats, peanuts and almonds.

Manganese RDA 1.2mg

Involved with enzyme function, including those involved with stabilising blood sugar. Helps form healthy bones, cartilage, cell tissues and nerves. Is essential for reproduction and red blood cell formation. Is required for neurological function.

Found in whole grains, leafy green vegetables, endive, lettuce, beetroot and celery.

Selenium RDA 900ug

Is an important antioxidant. It boosts the immune system, helping to fight and prevent infections, slows down ageing, promotes energy, and helps prevent arthritis, cancer and arteriosclerosis. Works with vitamin E.

Found in brewer's yeast, raw wheatgerm, tuna, molasses, herrings, cottage cheese, cabbage, courgettes, beef liver, cod and chicken.

Iodine RDA 220ug

Is essential for thyroid hormone synthesis. It raises the metabolic rate, prevents the accumulation of cholesterol and improves the quality of coat, skin, claws and teeth. It helps regulate the way cells use oxygen, promoting energy production and improves mental functions. Is important for growth and development of puppies.

Found in kelp, shellfish and seaweeds. Vegetables of the brassica family, i.e. cabbage, kale, brussel sprouts etc contain an ingredient that inhibits the absorption of iodine and should not be fed at the same time as foods or supplements containing iodine. Iodine should **not** be given where there is an under active thyroid problem.

Roughage

Roughage or dietary fibre is indigestible matter and herein lies its value as it enables the muscles of the alimentary canal to propel food through the system maintaining a clean colon free from unfriendly bacteria.

Fresh vegetables, fruit, whole grains and legumes provide all the naturally occurring types of fibre. High fibre vegetables include celery, leafy green, broccoli, spinach carrots and apple.

Absence of roughage is likely to lead to constipation and its attendant disorders. Dietary fibre provides bulk and many are able to absorb several times their own weight in water. Always make sure that there is a constant supply of fresh water as if not enough is drunk problems may be aggravated.

How much?

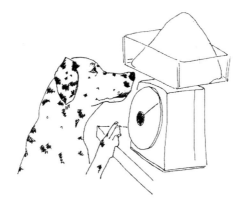

Now we have seen what your dog needs in his diet, we must look at how much should he eat to meet his requirements.

Each dog has individual needs that are governed by size, metabolic rate, work load (how much exercise, both mental and physical) and the conditions he lives in. If you had two ostensibly identical dogs, living in the same conditions, doing the same workload you would find that their dietary needs would be different. You know your dog better than anyone and can soon see which foods suit him and keep him in peak condition. By this we mean that your dog is active without losing weight or prone to building up a reserve of surplus fat.

There is a primeval urge in dogs to eat whenever there is an opportunity and thus store for the hypothetical rainy day. For most dogs this rainy day won't arrive so do not be fooled when your dog tries to tell you he needs more food – he almost can't help himself. He may be greedy but he almost certainly won't be hungry. Therefore when you have arrived at the optimum amount to feed your dog, keep to it. Any treats or rewards must be taken into account when feeding the daily ration.

The following table is a guide to how much you should feed your dog. Remember you know your dog best and can make adjustments to suit the individual dog. There are many, many theories on the optimum diet for the adult dog. Most breeders are convinced that their regime is correct for the particular breed but no two will be the same. Older nutritional tables suggest a greater calorific intake, usually about 15%. Whether this is because the dog of fifty years ago took more exercise and often lived in an unheated kennel, so needing more energy, or they were just fatter is hard to say. What is important is that your dog is fed a diet that suits him, meets all his nutritional requirements and fits in with your daily routine and household budget. Regard this table as a starting point and make adjustments where necessary.

Weight of dog in lb

	10lb	30lb	50lb	70lb	90lb
Puppies	990	-----	-----	-----	-----
For Maintenance	296	674	989	1,270	1,550

Weight of dog in lb

	10lb	30lb	50lb	70lb	90lb
For Moderate Work	404	922	1,353	1,740	2,100
For Hard Work	748	1,380	2,100	2,450	3,050

Pregnant dogs need about 25% greater calorific intake.

Young active dogs need about 10% more calories.

Older active dogs need about 20% less calories.

There are some schools of thought that advocate even less calories. Use your eyes. If you can easily feel but not see the ribs of your dog and there is a waist when viewed from above, an abdominal tuck when viewed from the side with no fat deposits over the back and base of the tail, then you've got it about right.

An 1862 book on dog care suggests the following way of judging the 'wholesome limit of your dogs appetite.' 'Give him an ample amount or more and keep your eye on him. If he is in health, he will set to and not abate his industry till he feels comfortably full, then he will raise his head and move away from the remnants. Marking this to save him eating to completion as he certainly will if allowed, you remove what is left and so learn what should be his regular allowance.' This is a useful way of deciding your dogs ration if he is about the right weight but the over weight or greedy dog will be capable of eating more than is good for him and the dog with poor digestion who needs several small meals throughout the day may not get enough. However, this is a useful way of determining the amount your dog is comfortable eating at one sitting.

You may wonder how you calculate calories if you are making your dog's food yourself. There are many books giving accurate calorie counts for all foods and if you read the packaging on most bought ingredients you will have a good idea, but for meat and fish that you may buy from a butcher or a fishmonger with no packaging, the following can be used as a rule of thumb.

Beef (varying with fat content)	50 – 100 per ounce
Chicken (without skin)	50 per ounce
Chicken (with skin)	75 per ounce
Lamb	70 per ounce
Liver	40 per ounce
Cod	53 per ounce
Haddock	20 per ounce
Herring	67 per ounce
Salmon	39 per ounce
Sardines (tinned)	84 per ounce
Butter	214 per ounce
Beef/lamb dripping	260 per ounce
Vegetable Oils	260 per ounce

Most green vegetables are low in calories and may be given freely. The important thing to remember is that the calories in the biscuit you use, the fat you may add in the form of oils, or the way the food is prepared will account for over half the calories given.

The companion dog often benefits from having his daily ration divided into two meals as his lifestyle does not give him the rest sufficient to digest one big meal.

Breakfast can be a thick slice of wholemeal bread, or some of the daily biscuit ration mixed with goats' milk. Twice a week, an egg may be substituted for the milk or porridge made with goats' milk may be given.

This gives the dog the energy to enjoy his exercise. Needless to say this meal should be given a minimum of one hour before any exercise. Dinner should be given when the dog has completed his exercise/work for the day and has plenty of time to digest his food. This meal will consist of the main protein content of the ration and the rest of the biscuit ration plus any vegetables and herbs you choose to give. The amount of protein required varies according to the amount of energy your dog expends – too much and you will have a hyperactive dog, too little and your dog will be fatigued and unable to maintain a healthy system. Again there are many studies into the optimum amount of protein that you should feed; the recommendations vary from ten to fifty percent by weight of the total daily ration. Start off by giving about a third of the daily total weight of food as meat and adjust accordingly.

Should your dog have stored too much fat, the best remedy is more exercise and fewer calories. There is a slimming pill being marketed and available from your vet but it is not recommended except in cases of morbid obesity. It is much better for the health of both dog and owner to get out, get fit and eat a little less.

Puppies have quite different needs to an adult dog. At first they need about twice the calorific intake per pound of bodyweight to an adult of the same breed. They require twice the amount of protein and half as much again of fat. They should be fed several times a day from the age of about four weeks when the mothers' milk is no longer providing all its needs. During this time, Mum herself will need extra calories (three to five times as much depending on the number of puppies) to provide for her pups. Giant breeds have proportionally smaller digestive tracts and may not be able to eat enough to sustain them and provide for their pups. Owners of such dogs may need to start feeding their puppies supplemental food at an early age. Take advice from your vet on this.

Older dogs need up to 20% less calories as they do less work and their metabolism slows down. The protein portion of the ration may need to be increased to maintain the protein reserves. As your dog ages monitor the weight level and make adjustments to the amount fed as necessary. Many older dogs become obese if they are given the same quantity of food as they were in their prime and this can seriously impair the quality of life of your dog as well as contributing to major diseases.

When dogs have been ill their energy requirements may increase, especially if the illness has led to a loss of appetite. Some illnesses require or will be helped by a special diet, your vet will advise in such cases

Having now learnt what a dog requires for optimum health, the question is how to ensure that our feeding regime covers all these requirements. In the following chapter we shall look at the different and often confusing regimes which all assure us that we are doing the best for our dogs.

Which regime?

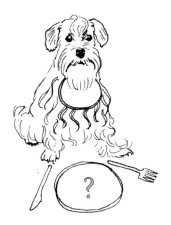

During 10,000 years or so of domestication the dog has shown great adaptability in deriving nourishment from foods not originally designed for his digestive tract. Behaviourist Steven Lindsay reminds us that 'a long history of domestication behaviourally segregates the wolf and the domestic dog and one must take care not to overly generalise between the two canids in terms of their response to motivation and behaviour.' The same applies to the feeding of the domestic dog. Just because he is descended from wild dogs doesn't mean that todays companion dog has the same nutritional needs or the same digestive system. Adaptions have taken place. Feral dogs scavenge and do not need to form a pack to survive – they have no need to hunt and probably couldn't. Necessity in lean times means that he has become virtually omnivorous, and a scavenger. This very ability to digest a wide variety of foods leads the digestive fluids to become habituated to dealing with certain foods in combination and any change can alter the balances whether it because the new food is too rich, too acid, too alkali, too sloppy or too concentrated. Wherever possible it is a good idea to get a dog used to a variety of foods when he is a puppy so that he does not become a fussy eater. His digestion can then become accustomed to and cope with all foods and maintain a wide intake of essential nutrients.

The first, and most important thing to be aware of is how our dog's digestive system works and thus reacts to change. Put simply a dog chews its food to enable swallowing. Unlike humans the alkaline saliva does not start the digestive process but facilitates passage to the stomach. Do not be alarmed if you think your dog seems to bolts its food with indecent haste. There is only need for concern if the speed of ingestion is such that the food is brought straight back up again, in which case give larger pieces or you can semi- freeze the meal so that it is more solid and requires chewing to break it down into swallowable size pieces. Once the food is in the stomach it is broken down into a broth like fluid and transmitted to the small intestine where it is rendered alkaline. The pancreas and glands lining the gut produce digestive enzymes which accelerate the rate at which insoluble compounds are rendered soluble and are available for absorption. The passage of food through the system is facilitated by the involuntary movement of the smooth muscles of the digestive tract with a churning movement that aids the absorption of all the energy giving nourishment, leaving only the indigestible residue to be passed to the large intestine where it is stored until it is voided as faeces. It is important to understand that once the digestive system is used to certain food stuffs, the proportions of enzymes and stomach acids can not be changed overnight without some disruptions. Any change in feeding patterns or foodstuffs must be done very slowly over a period of a week to ten days as sudden change can result in massive upsets which can take weeks to put right. If you are changing a food start by adding 10% of the new food to 90% of the amount of food you usually give. Carry on this 10% substitution every other day until you are giving 100% of the new food. This particularly applies to changes in commercial foods but can also apply to raw or homemade diets.

What type of food should you be feeding your dog? There are pros and cons in any feeding regime and we shall now discuss them.

Commercial Foods

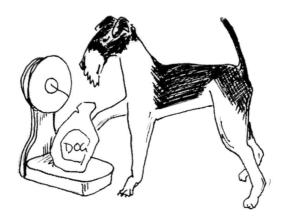

Most dogs are fed commercial varieties. Try to ensure that the ingredients are good quality. Some foods use mechanically reclaimed meat or meat derivatives, sweepings from human food production, strange colourings to make the food look attractive (to you, not your dog) and artificial smells to make it attractive to the dog.

One of the biggest worries is the preservatives used, these are often not even listed but come under the blanket heading of E. U. permitted. These are used to try and prevent the oils and fats from going rancid but can have many ill effects. If the preservatives are not listed ring or write to the manufacturer for a full list of ingredients.

The first thing to look at in any commercial food is the ingredients, bear in mind these are listed in descending order, the highest volume ingredient is listed first. The first thing to look for is whether the first listed ingredient is an animal based protein. The entire protein content should be at the head of the list. Avoid foods that list by-products and food fractions e.g. wheat middlings or corn gluten rather than whole grains, these products are left overs from human food processing and don't provide the best nutrition. Look for natural preservatives such as vitamin C (ascorbic acid) and vitamin E and mixed Tocopherols. Avoid foods containing Ethoxquin, BHA/BHT (found in North American pet foods but banned in Europe) and Propylene Glycol. Flavour enhancers such as Phosphoric acid and artificial colouring agents such as Azo ozodyes, and Sodium Nitrate should also be avoided. Look for foods that contain Essential Fatty Acids and additional antioxidants such as vitamins C, E and flavanoids.

Recently there has been a huge scandal in North America as the contents of some brands of both dry and canned dog food has been proved to be responsible for a large number of animal deaths. One culprit has made an acknowledgement that internal testing procedures were at fault allowing corn tainted with a mould called aflatoxin, which causes liver damage, to contaminate the production lines. Another recall in 2007 was due to the addition of melamine in certain brands that had been produced in China. As a result of these incidents the FDA is taking steps to develop ingredient, processing and labelling standards to improve the safety of pet foods.

There are no such proposals in the UK at present but keep pestering the individual manufactures and the Pet Food Manufacturers Association for details of the source of the ingredients and the preservatives used and your concerns about possible toxic side effects and maybe they will follow their American counterparts.

Complete Foods

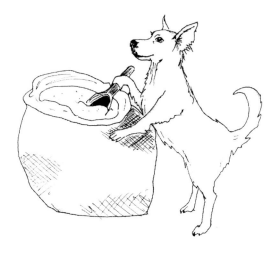

Complete foods are very widely used, largely because of their convenience; you can buy in bulk, one scoop and a bowl of water and job done. However are you sure your dog is getting a balanced diet? A complete food? Complete for which dog? You can't adjust the protein/vegetable requirements to suit the level of work and the metabolism of your dog – it's all in one. Problems arise when this type of food is topped up with meat and or vegetables to make it less boring, then the nutritional balance is completely disrupted.

Once the manufacturer has calculated the formulas for their offering the ingredients are mixed together and ground by hammer mill to a suitably small size from whence they are fed into an extruder where the ground mix is converted to pellets of various shapes and sizes.

During the extrusion process, steam or water are added and the dough like mixture heated so that the starches in the cereal component of the mix are gelatinised which holds all the ingredients together in one homogenous form. This cooking process also ensures that the starches are rendered more easily digestible so that their full potential to supply energy is achieved.

The dough is then forced through the die plate of the mill. Considerable pressure is generated by this process, so much so, that the difference between the inside of the machine and the normal atmosphere causes the composition to pop as the dough comes through the die developing a texture that is easily digested.

The extruded pellets contain roughly 25 – 30 % moisture which is removed by baking. This allows for storage for long periods as all the moisture has been removed, preventing any bacterial or fungal growth. The final stage is to spray hot fat, mixed with preservatives and flavourings on to the pellets to make them look and smell appetising and able to be stored for long periods.

The protein content in dry foods is either from animal origin or oil seed / vegetable origin.

Those proteins from animal origins are often the residues of muscle meat, which due to production methods can contain a good proportion of bone which is rich in calcium and phosphorus. Too much calcium can lead to malabsorption or destruction of minerals, the most important being copper which can lead to skin problems. The other main source of protein is the residue from the dressing of carcasses at the abattoir and is what is classified as unfit for human consumption. This is much lower in calcium and protein but higher in fats. Some manufacturers raise the protein by adding dried blood, while others mix the different sources.

Fish and poultry content are usually produced by the same process, i.e. the remnants of human food processing or industrial applications. Some of the vegetable content is provided by the residues of oil seed extraction process. Additives (vitamins and essential amino acids) are added in sufficient quantities to ensure that the loss due to heat damage in processing still leaves the required amounts in the final product.

Canned Foods

Canned dog food has become known as wet food for good reason, – many are 70% water. Manufacturers now state the water content so read the label and you may be surprised to find that you are paying for very expensive water.

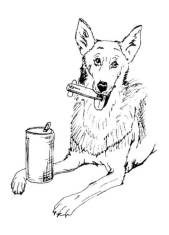

The ingredients are sourced and manufactured in much the same way as complete foods but instead of getting dried pellets you get a more moist food. The meat content in wet foods is usually no more than 4 or 5%. Check the label to ensure that there is actually a real meat content, some times those inviting chunks are not real meat but Soya or other cereals which are often used as filler. If you are feeding wet food with biscuit or dehydrated mixer the carbohydrate content of your dogs diet is likely to be far higher than you would imagine or want to give. That said though, it is undesirable to feed canned food without biscuit or mixer as the hard biscuit provides work for the teeth and gums as well as essential fibre and roughage.

Pet food labels do not generally list essential ingredients by weight but must state the minimum percentage of crude protein and fat and the maximum crude filler and moisture content. In this instance crude refers to the testing method. It is quite easy to work out the actual content by using the following formula:

crude percentage x weight of daily portion

e.g. if you give a 454 gm can per day and it contains 8% crude protein the sum would be 0.08 x 454 =36.3 therefore you are giving 36.3 gms of protein.

Although convenient, there are drawbacks in that your dog's digestive system very quickly becomes adapted to his usual food so if you regularly use a particular brand you may have repercussions if you change to a different manufacturer. Variety helps the system deal with a wide range of foods.

The Bone and Raw Food Diet

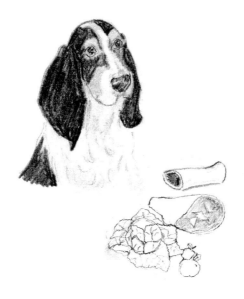

The raw food diet is growing in popularity and has much to recommend it as it attempts to replicate the wild dog's diet. By natural disposition the dog is a flesh eating hunter, his teeth are designed not for the modern starch and cellulose diet but for tearing and ripping meat from the bones of prey which exercises the teeth and gums and checks the deposit of tartar, which nowadays is all too frequently seen, leading to loss of teeth and or frequent dental operations.

The advantages of this diet are that the preservative problem is overcome, your dog will have cleaner teeth, mental stimulation and a time-consuming hobby as he chews his bones. By feeding your dog this diet you are in control and can ensure he is receiving high quality whole foods as you are buying the ingredients.

Your butcher can be very helpful in providing bones and offcuts but do be aware of how much fat is being given. Frozen raw meat is available from some pet shops, but again take care to check the fat levels. The proportion of lites should also be monitored as although hearts, lungs and other offal are good for your dog they should not be fed every day as this will lead to an excess of vitamin A.

The combinations of foodstuffs are vitally important in this type of diet. Too many bones can lead to constipation or even hernia. Excessive calcium can also cause mineral imbalances as we have previously discussed.

Too much protein can be a problem in the unbalanced diet, this can lead to kidney diseases and often to behavioural problems.

When meaty bones are fed it is important to feed the right type of bone which under no circumstances should be cooked. Cooking makes bones brittle and liable to splinter, and the heat of cooking destroys vital nutrients. Large shin bones are too hard even for big dogs – teeth can be chipped and jaws can be strained. Your butcher can split these bones length ways so that the marrow can be licked out but the density of the bone means that you should be cautious in the amount of chewing you should allow. Small dogs should be given bones commensurate with their size, start off giving bendy chicken wings and progress to whole carcases. Lamb shoulder bones are also suitable. Rib bones are good but care must be taken to ensure that your dog does not get these bones caught in his teeth or in the mouth. For this reason give bones when you are around to deal with any such problems. Also care must be taken not to give your dog too many bones as an excess can lead to constipation and hernia, or, in some cases, kidney damage as a result of too much calcium.

In this type of diet raw meaty bones make up about 60% of the food given. They are usually given in the mornings and the rest of the diet in the evenings. It is worth remembering that raw meat is more stimulative than cooked meat.

When feeding in the wild dogs get the vegetable portion of their diet from the guts and stomach of their prey. This vegetable matter is semi-digested and this makes it easy for the dog to absorb the nutrients as a dogs digestive system is not geared up for digesting cellulose. The fermentation in the gut of the prey breaks down the cellulose into glucose and fatty acids. This frees the carbohydrates and proteins in a form that the dog's digestive system can easily deal with. To gain full nutritional benefits from the vegetables we feed, we need to mimic the contents of a herbivore's stomach and intestines. We do this by pulping the vegetables in a food processor or old-fashioned mincer. Some people like to use a juicer and give the pulp and pour some of the juice in to the dogs meal but some juices are very bitter and thus unpalatable. It is important to feed a variety of vegetables so that a wide range of nutrients is given. A word of warning, go easy on the cabbage family – excessive amounts can lead to unpleasant wind problems even though cabbage in moderation is very healing for gut problems.

Other foodstuffs such as eggs and cheese can also be given; we discuss these in the next chapter.

If you are interested in feeding a raw food diet there are many books outlining in greater detail how to do it. The most well known is 'Give Your Dog a Bone' by Dr Ian Billinghurst

The Home Prepared Diet

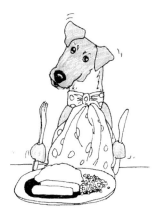

By preparing your dog's diet yourself you can overcome many of the concerns we have talked about in regard to commercial foods. If you source the ingredients that you use to feed your dog you can be sure that the quality is as good as possible and that there are no strange additives. The only preservative you will need is a freezer.

As we have learnt, it is important to give a variety of foods that ensure a wide range of vitamin and mineral intake and that can contribute to a robust digestion. With a little thought and organisation this need not be a complicated business. Many of the aspects of the raw food diet are the same but some people are unhappy with the idea of bones or chunks of raw meat being dragged around their house or being buried in their gardens. There is also the concern that raw meat and bones may contain parasites and bacteria harmful to their dogs and other members of the family, particularly where there are small children present, so some people prefer to cook the meat element of their pets' food for hygiene reasons. Hard biscuits can be as good a teeth cleaner as bones. If you follow the basic biscuit recipe and shape the dough into a thick sausage shape or if you are feeling creative, a bone shape, the chewing and gnawing will help remove the build up of plaque and tartar.

If you want to prepare your dog's diet yourself, do not think that you have to provide a balanced meat and two veg meal every day. Variety is the name of the game and as long as the diet is balanced over the course of a week all will be well and your dog will look forward to his meals rather than be faced with the same 'stew' everyday.

Where the meat is cooked it should be done as lightly as possible, grilled, baked or simmered with a little water. Fried food is as unhealthy for our dogs as it is for us. Sufficient quantity for two or three days may be prepared at one time and stored in the fridge. Larger quantities may be divided into daily portions and frozen. Do remember to clearly mark the food you have prepared (for your dog) as it is incredibly annoying to find that you've just defrosted your prize casserole for the dog. Chicken and fish are excellent additions to the diet. They are easily digested, low in fat and contain minerals, essential fats and acids. Chicken is an easily digested protein. It is particularly useful when your dog is unwell, a soup made from fresh chicken stock contains T cells which aid the healing process and can often be tolerated when little else can. If you have a cooked chicken for supper do not throw the carcass away but make a strong stock by boiling until the liquid goes to jelly when cooled, strain and use either for soups or gravies for yourself or as part of your dog's meal. Fish is also good for your dog. White fish is light and low in fat but the inclusion of oily fish, mackerel, sardine, tuna, herring or salmon is essential once or twice a week as it is a major source of omega 3 and omega 6. These essential fatty acids are required for the function of every cell, tissue, gland and organ. Lites, that is liver, heart, kidney, brain and lungs are very rich in minerals and vitamins especially the B vitamins. Regular inclusion in the diet contributes to healthy skin, temperament (because of the B vitamins) and blood. Organ food is very rich so small amounts are given, it is often cooked as some dogs find it easier to digest this way and cooking will kill any parasites present if you have obtained it from a source other than that suitable for human consumption. If you want to feed raw offal it is advisable to source it from a butcher.

Pork meat is often seen in commercial foods but not very much is fed to dogs in raw or home produced diets. This is because that whilst pork is a good source of protein and minerals it is low in most vitamins except the B vitamins. Many dogs find large amounts of pork indigestible and when it is cooked the cholesterol level rises significantly as some cuts can be high in fat. If you want to feed pork do so cautiously, ensure your dog's system can cope, and remember to feed extra vitamin containing foods.

Tripe is a useful addition to the diet, but it must be uncleaned (green) tripe as it provides a natural way of ingesting vegetable matter.

Dogs can not live on meat alone so this meat dish needs to be mixed with a proportion of good quality additive-free biscuit. There are now a number of small manufacturers making such a product or you can make your own, the recipe section tells you how. Pasta and rice may be given but only in small quantities as they have little real food value unless they are of the wholewheat or brown variety. They are pure carbohydrate, which your dog only needs in small quantities and the excess is likely to head straight to his waistline. If you feed either pasta or rice it should be no more than once a week and should proportionally replace the biscuit element otherwise you may find that such a high carbohydrate meal will result in a very energetic dog. Meat trimmings from your own cooking can be used provided they are not too fatty. The same rule applies to left overs which can form a good basis to your dog's meal. It is economical and saves waste as long as the following provisos are met. They are that the fat content should be minimal, there should be very little if any salt and no onions included. French onion soup no matter how nutritious for humans is one left over dish that should never be given to your dog.

Vegetables are a welcome addition to the meal as they are a rich source of vitamins, minerals, enzymes, anti oxidants and soluble fibre. If you have left over green veg include them but starchy vegetables such as potatoes and some root vegetables should be given in minimum quantities. Some would say avoid them altogether but dogs like potatoes and the odd one or two as a treat will do no harm. Raw vegetables are obviously the most nutritious and we have discussed how to prepare and feed them in the previous section. The lists of vitamins and minerals will guide you as to the contents of various vegetables but the ones I have found to be most easily accepted are as follows (do remember that dogs are individuals and their tastes may vary).

Broccoli, carrots, green peas, green beans, cabbage, spinach lettuce and parsley. Broccoli should not be give if there is a thyroid problem. Spinach should be avoided where there is a kidney problem and cabbage can cause flatulence.

Eggs and dairy produce have their place in a balanced, varied diet. Eggs are a great source of protein, sulphur, magnesium and lecithin. They contain lots of minerals, vitamins and essential fatty acids and are very easy to digest. They may be given raw or mixed with a little milk or crushed vegetable or occasionally even a little cheese. Scrambled eggs are very binding and can be useful in cases of upset stomachs and diahorrea.

Dogs love cheese and a little is good for them as a source of protein but it usually has a high fat and salt content. Indeed it is just dried out, fermented milk which is not awfully good for some dogs as they find it hard to digest. It is probably a good idea to save cheese as a treat or a training reward. Cottage cheese however is good in moderation as it is highly digestible and a great source of Trytophan, which converted into serotonin relieves nervousness and depression. However cheese and cottage cheese are **not** recommended for dogs with heart problems because of the sodium content

In a varied diet a milk meal may be included every so often. This is when you would mix raw egg or cheese and maybe a little oil with the usual biscuit or mixer. Raw milk is of course preferable but can be difficult to obtain. It is now becoming more readily available at farmers markets or at the farm gate of some organic farms. At present it is still illegal for supermarkets to sell it.

Yogurt is indispensable in the dog's diet and should be included regularly. It is easily digested and helps fortify the intestinal flora.

It is particularly beneficial in cases of upset stomach and when antibiotics have been given. Both cows' and goats' yogurt are readily available.

Goats' milk is often better tolerated than cows' milk as it is more easily digested, particularly by young animals. It is very useful for putting condition on ill or run down dogs but because of its richness it is best given diluted by up to 50% water.

Soya milk is to be avoided as it is too hard for dogs to digest and has a poor amino acid profile.

Herbs, Spices and Supplements

Most herbs and spices can be incorporated into your dog's diet. If you are using either in your own cooking sprinkle a little over your dog's meal as they are rich in minerals and oils that can play a part in the overall wellbeing of your pet. They all have medicinal as well as culinary uses and these can be very useful in many illnesses. There are many good herbals available but if using herbs in therapeutic quantities be guided by a qualified herbalist or discuss herbs as a form of treatment with your vet. Well intentioned home diagnosis or home medication can cause more problems than they solve.

Honey is a great addition to the diet and also has many healing properties. Being anti-inflammatory, antibacterial, antifungal and antiseptic it may be used as a healing agent in minor cuts and sores as well as providing protection if given orally. Two or three teaspoonfuls on a regular basis can work wonders. Manuka honey has the highest anti bacterial action and is often successfully used in hospital to treat stubborn leg ulcers.

Ideally, supplements should be unnecessary and in many cases, if you pay attention to your dog's diet, they are. However, in these days of intensive farming many soils are depleted of essential nutrients as the fertilisers used are often specific to the crops to be grown rather than providing a broad spectrum of minerals and trace elements. If you feel that the food you and your dog eat is grown on tired overworked soil then supplementation may be in order. Some people advocate a daily dose and some think that there should be no supplementation at all. Consider what you are feeding your dog and the state of his health. There are expensive tests available but use your common sense, for instance if you are giving oily fish once or twice a week then there are probably sufficient EFAs in the diet, but if your dog doesn't like fish then supplementation may be beneficial. If you decide to supplement, a multi mineral, multi vitamin and essential fatty acids would be the place to start as they will provide the right balance of the different nutrients. Try supplementing for a couple of months and decide if there is any improvement to your dog's overall health, then leave them for a period. You may have corrected any deficiencies and to supplement further would upset the balance in the opposite direction. Remember anything in excess is a poison. Therapeutic doses can be very effective in correcting a number of illnesses but these must be given under the supervision of a qualified nutritionalist. Always discuss the situation with your vet to ensure the supplements you are giving do not exacerbate the condition and interact beneficially with prescribed medicines.

Kelp can be a useful addition to the diet as it contains an abundance of minerals and trace elements, the most prized being iodine, which can be difficult to include in a dog's diet. Iodine helps the thyroid gland function properly through the production of thyroxine. It raises the metabolic rate, helping to burn excess fat preventing the accumulation of cholesterol which helps stabilize body weight. It calms nerves and contributes to healthy coat, skin, claws and teeth. It is also believed to reduce the risk of some cancers. Kelp is harvested from a variety of cold water seaweeds, dried and sold in tablet or powder form. Some health food shops now sell several varieties of dried seaweed which can be incorporated in the diet.

Spirulina is an algae that is harvested from warm alkaline lakes such as Lake Chad in Africa and Lake Texcoco in Mexico. It is a versatile food supplement which strengthens the immune system and increases resistance to disease and inflammation. Spirulina contains over 65% complete protein which is so well balanced that it is easier to digest than meat. It contains many minerals including potassium, calcium, zinc, magnesium, manganese, selenium, iron and phosphorus. It is also a rich source of the B vitamins, vitamin E, beta carotene, GLA and chlorophyll. For these reasons it is a very useful supplement when your dog is recovering from illness or is under the weather. It is available from health food shops in powder and tablet form.

Brewer's yeast contains excellent concentrations of the B vitamins including B12 and is up to 45% protein, containing 17 amino acids including all the essential ones. It is a rich source of minerals and trace elements. There are many types of brewer's yeast, depending on what the yeast has been grown on, so read the labels. Those that are grown on selinium salts provide a great source of selenium that is very easily absorbed. Brewer's yeast is available from health food counters in tablet, flake or powder form. It is useful as a supplement where there is poor diet or illness. As it is a yeast, initially brewer's yeast should only be given in very small quantities as it may cause indigestion and bloating. This will subside gradually as the digestive system becomes accustomed to the yeast. If there is an underlying fungal infection brewer's yeast should not be given. Calcium should be given with high intakes of yeast as it helps balance the phosphorus levels.

Garlic, although a member of the onion family, is often used to combat fleas and internal parasites. It is anti bacterial, anti fungal and antithrombic and will help boost the immune system. Those who choose to use it give a small raw clove two or three times a week and many swear they are never troubled by fleas. If you give too much garlic you will have a very pungent dog and in excess it can cause stomach upsets. One of the best ways to give it is to include it in a meal that is lightly cooked. Remember garlic and dairy products do not go together.

What your dog does not need

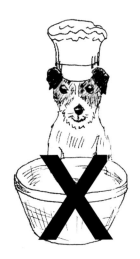

There are few foodstuffs that are poisonous to dogs but **the following should be avoided at all costs:**

- Avocado
- Chocolate
- Elderberry
- Grapes and raisins
- Green tomato
- Rhubarb especially the leaves
- Onions
- Leeks
- Citrus fruits.

There may be other foods that your dog, as an individual, is allergic to so, if you think that any particular food is having a detrimental effect, remove it from the diet and see if things improve. If you dog shows any signs of severe allergic reaction or symptoms of poisoning i.e. vomiting, diarrhoea, panting, unsteadiness or dehydration consult your vet immediately.

There are many plants that your dog may come across in the garden, on his walk, or even around the house that may prove to be poisonous. As a general rule it is a good idea to stop your dog eating strange plants, digging up your flowerbeds and eating bulbs, or playing with unidentified plant matter. Do not use cocoa based mulches on your garden. They can be as deadly as chocolate. Many garden centres now label poisonous plants and comprehensive lists are available from various publishers but the main ones to be on the look out for are:

- Aconite
- Amaryllis
- Azalea
- Bluebell
- Buttercup
- Calla Lily
- Clematis
- Cyclamen
- Daffodil bulbs
- Easter Lily

- English Ivy
- Foxglove
- Geranium
- Holly Berries
- Honeysuckle
- Hyacinth bulbs
- Lily of the Valley
- Mistletoe
- Nightshade
- Philodendron of any type
- Poinsettia
- Ragwort
- Rhododendron
- Rhubarb leaves
- Swiss Cheese plants
- Yew
- Wisteria
- Any foodstuff that contains the artificial sweetner xylitol which can be deadly.

In Conclusion

We have seen that there are many feeding regimes available to dog owners and outlined the advantages and disadvantages each offers. Whichever one you choose make sure the ingredients are sourced as naturally as possible. Read the labels and work out exactly what you are giving your dog to eat. See if it can be improved by adding variety and fresh foods. Your dog is unique and his requirements are individual. Note what his likes and dislikes are, and use this to your advantage. Favourites can be used as a training reward but don't give too much too often or it won't be a treat. There have been cases where dogs have been fed so much chicken that they now refuse it under all circumstances. If your dog refuses a particular food it is probably with good reason, he knows that it doesn't agree with him. If you are introducing an unfamiliar food do it slowly as we have discussed. If he still refuses it listen to him and remove it from his diet.

Well-being and vitality are a result of more than just good quality food, exercise and comfortable quarters. The zest for life we so appreciate in our dogs comes from their living in a nurturing environment where they are loved and involved in family life. Isolation however comfortable is distressing for most dogs, they need to be part of a social group ... their family.

Grooming is an important part of maintaining the overall health of your dog. A daily brush keeps the coat clean, it is important to remove the dead hair as this will stimulate the blood supply to the skin, encourage new growth and result in less dog hairs around the house. Last, but not least, grooming reinforces the bond between the dog and his owner. Most dogs like to be brushed and enjoy the contact time that grooming provides.

If you take an holistic approach to your dog's care and provide good food, water, warmth and lots of love you will have a happy and contented companion for many years.

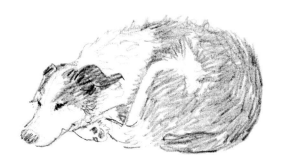

Recipes

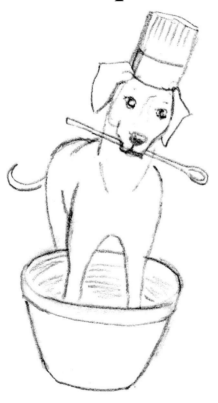

Recipes

In the some of the following recipes stock may be used instead of water, but home made or supermarket real stock is preferable to stock cubes as they have an incredibly high salt content and some contain preservatives. If you want to use stock cubes make a very weak mixture.

Malt extract is used as a sweetener in place of sugar. Very little is needed to give an equivalent sweetness and it is packed full of minerals. Dogs love the smell and find it very appetising.

Basic Biscuits

These biscuits may be used as meal or mixer with the main meal. They keep well in an air tight container and so may be made in fairly large quantities. These can be very economical if baked when you are using the oven for family cooking.

2 lb Wholemeal flour
4 oz (scant ¼ pint) sunflower or other vegetable oil
Water or stock

Mix the flour and oil as you would pastry, when the oil is evenly distributed add enough water to make a stiff dough. Don't worry if you add too much water just add more flour little by little until you have the required consistency. Roll out the dough to about ¼ inch thick and then take a knife and score the dough into approx ¼ inch squares, (smaller for puppies and small dogs).

Place on a baking tray and bake at the bottom of a moderate oven gas mark 5/300ºF/190ºC until quite dry. Allow to cool in the oven. When cool store in an airtight container. This dough can also be shaped into thicker bone or sausage shapes, baked for a slightly longer period, and then given as a bone substitute.

Meat Biscuits

These are a favourite and very economical as the fat content can be obtained from your own cooking. If you have a roast, or lamb chops save the fat that you would normally pour off and use in these biscuits

2 lb Wholemeal flour
4 oz fat
Water or water and any left over gravy or stock

Warm the fat, work it into the flour and proceed as above.

Suet Biscuits

If you haven't any animal fat to hand and want to make a tasty biscuit your can use beef suet which can be bought ready prepared. Vegetable suet is available but doesn't seem so palatable.

2 lb flour
5 oz suet
1 teaspoon baking powder
Cold water

Add the baking powder to the dry flour, mix well, add the suet, and mix together with sufficient cold water to form a dough. Proceed as above or make small balls about the size of your thumb and place on the baking tray. When cooked and cooled, store in an airtight container.

Oat Biscuits

Oats are gluten free, so are useful where there is a gluten intolerance. They are valuable from a nutritional standpoint as they have much the same profile as wheat but with more biotin and fat. They release energy slowly so are a sustaining food.

½ lb fine/medium oatmeal
½ lb coarse oatmeal
4 oz wholemeal flour
3 oz fat of your choice (use different fats for different flavours)
Boiling water or stock

Place the oatmeal in a bowl. Melt the fat in about ¼ pint of boiling water and pour over the oatmeal which should be just covered. If you need more water add extra. Allow to stand for 20 to 30 minutes so that the water is absorbed, top up if necessary. When the mixture is cool enough to handle start adding the wholemeal flour until you have a firm dough and turn out on to a well floured board. Roll out to the desired thickness and cut to shape. Place biscuits on a greased baking tray. Cook in a preheated oven Gas mark 4/350ºF/180ºC. Allow to cool in the oven. Store in an airtight container.

Oat Crunchies

2 oz whole (Jumbo) oats
2 oz porridge oats
3 oz vegetable oil or butter
2 tablespoons malt extract
A baking tin approx 11 x 7 inches.

Gently melt the malt extract and the oil in a saucepan. Do not let it burn. Pour the mixture over the oats and stir until everything is coated and well mixed. Turn the mixture into a lightly greased baking tin. Place in the centre of a preheated oven Gas mark 5, 375°F/190°C for 15 minutes. Remove from the oven, and when it has cooled slightly but is still warm cut the mixture into desired size. Allow to cool completely before storing in an airtight container.

Treats and Rewards

These are special delights that your dog earns for good behaviour. Most are richer than everyday foods so should be used judiciously. They do not form part of the general diet but account must be taken when giving the daily ration as too many rich treats can upset the balance and result in weight gain.

Cheese Biscuits

1 lb wholemeal flour
2 oz vegetable oil or butter
2 oz hard cheese finely grated
1 egg, and cold water to mix

Rub the butter or oil into the flour, add the grated cheese. Mix the egg with a little water and add to the flour to form a stiff dough. Roll out and cut into desired size and shape.

Bake in a moderately hot oven Gas mark 4/350ºF/180ºC for about 15–20 minutes and allow to cool in the oven.

Very Rich Cheese Biscuits

You can eat these too! They are jolly useful for party nibbles, but dogs love them and they are a great reward when training an activity your dog finds difficult.

2 oz wholemeal flour
2 oz grated cheddar cheese
2 oz grated red Leicester cheese
2 oz butter (you can use vegetable oil if you prefer)
Pinch of salt

Combine all the ingredients together in a bowl. Rub the mixture to the crumbly stage and then bring it together so that you have a pastry. If the mixture is too dry you can add a little water or milk, but you probably won't need to.

Roll out the dough to about 1/8th of an inch and cut to your desired shape. Put on a greased baking tray in the top of the oven at gas mark 5/375ºF/190ºC for 10–12 minutes. Remove from the oven and cool on a wire rack. Store in an airtight container.

Carrot Biscuits

1 large carrot weighing approx 3oz
8 oz Wholemeal flour
1 tablespoon malt extract
2 oz fat or oil
1 egg
1 teaspoon baking powder

Grate the carrot and put it in a mixing bowl with the wholemeal flour and the baking powder. Gently warm the malt extract with the oil until it is runny and pour into the bowl with the carrot and flour. Mix well then add the beaten egg, pour the batter into a baking tin and bake in the centre of the oven at gas mark 3/325ºF/170ºC for 25 mins. Cool on a rack and store in an air tight container.

A very easy method is just to tip all the ingredients into the bowl of a food processor, blitz for a few seconds until every thing is mixed together, and then pour into the baking tray.

Cheese and Spinach Pretzels

8 oz wholemeal flour
2 oz dried milk
4 oz grated cheddar or other hard cheese
5 oz chopped cooked spinach
4 tablespoons vegetable oil

Cook and drain the spinach, allow to cool. Squeeze as much water as possible from the cooked spinach and place in the bowl of the food processor. Add the grated cheese and the vegetable oil. Mix thoroughly but be careful not to over do it and make a puree. Put the bowl and contents in the fridge for about an hour. When the mixture is quite cold and has stiffened take it out of the fridge and add the flour and the dried milk and mix to a dough. Turn out on to a floured board and roll out to about ¼ inch and cut into desired shapes. You can make a sausage about the thickness of a pencil and make traditional pretzel shapes if you are feeling creative but it's a bit of a fiddle and quite frankly your dog won't care what shape his treat comes in. Cook on a lightly greased baking tray in the centre of the oven at gas mark 2/300ºF/150ºC for 40–45 minutes.

Peanut Butter Biscuits

These are very easy and very popular. Always use smooth peanut butter if giving to puppies.

8 oz wholemeal flour
2 oz peanut butter
Water

Rub the peanut butter into the flour. Using a food processor is fine if you prefer and is less sticky on your hands. Add a little water to form a dough, cut into desired shape and bake in the centre of the oven for 25 minutes at gas mark 4/350ºF./180ºC Allow to cool in the oven. Store in an airtight container.

Rich and Crumbly Peanut Butter Biscuits

8 oz wholemeal flour
4 oz oatmeal
2 oz malt extract
1 tablespoon of peanut oil or any vegetable oil
3 oz smooth peanut butter
1 teaspoon baking powder

A food processor is easier for this one. Combine all the ingredients in the bowl and mix until everything is amalgamated. Add some water a tablespoon at a time until you have nice dough. If you add too much water don't worry, stiffen the mixture with extra flour. Using a spoon or your fingers make golf ball sized balls, flatten them to approximately

¼ inch, place on a baking tray in the centre of the oven and cook at gas mark 3/275ºF/140ºC for 20 minutes. Allow to cool in the oven and then store in an airtight container.

Doggy Parkin

6 oz medium oatmeal
3 oz self raising wholemeal flour
4 oz malt extract
3 oz butter or margarine
1½ teaspoons dried ginger or 1 inch fresh ginger peeled and finely grated
1 small egg beaten
1 dessertspoon milk

Put the malt extract and the fat in a saucepan and heat gently until the extract is runny and the fat melted. At the same time put the dry ingredients in a bowl and mix together with a pinch of salt. Add this to the warm malt extract mixture and stir until everything is well blended. Now add the beaten egg and the milk. You should now have a batter like mixture that you pour into the prepared tin. Bake in the centre of the oven at gas mark 1/275ºF/140ºC for 1½ hours. Cool in the tin before turning out and storing. This may well sag in the middle but the dogs won't mind.

Liver

Liver is rich in many vitamins and minerals and most dogs love it. Liver can be very rich so making treats is an ideal way of including it in your dogs diet on a regular basis without causing stomach upsets.

Liver Jerky

This is the easiest of all the treat recipes as you don't actually do very much. It can be cooked at the same time as you are using the oven for another dish. Make small quantities to maintain freshness or if you want to make a larger batch it can be frozen.

Take your piece of liver, any type will do, pat it dry with kitchen paper, rub a little oil on the surface and place on a baking tray. Place in the bottom of the oven at gas mark 1/275ºF/140ºC and bake until it resembles shoe leather. Cool and cut into small squares and store in the fridge.

Liver Biscuits

1 lb wholemeal flour
2 oz liver
2 oz fat

In a food processor or liquidiser, place the liver, fat, and two tablespoons of water. Pulverise until you have a sloppy mixture. Add the flour and mix until everything is gathered into a firm dough. If you need to add more water do so a little at a time. Turn out on to a floured board, roll out to about ¼ inch thick and then score into suitable sized squares. Another way is to roll out into thin sausages which when cooked are convenient for breaking into treat sized pieces. Bake in the centre of the oven at gas mark 3/325ºF/170ºC for 1 hour or until hard. Allow to cool in the oven.

Liver Buns

2 oz liver
8 oz wholemeal flour
3 oz fat
2 eggs
1 ½ teaspoons baking powder.
½ tablespoon peas
½ tablespoon chopped carrots
½ tablespoon chopped beans
12 bun cases

Lightly cook half the liver and chop into small pieces, reserve. Blanch the vegetables for 3 minutes, cool and reserve. If you want to use frozen vegetables this makes life easy as they do not need blanching. Mix the flour and the baking powder well and then rub in the fat. In a food processor or liquidiser beat the eggs with the remaining raw liver until you have a smooth mixture. Add the cooked chopped liver and the vegetables. Fold the flour and fat mixture into the eggs and liver adding a little milk if necessary to get a dropping consistency. Divide the mixture equally between the paper bun cases. Put the filled bun cases into a bun tray and place on the shelf above the centre in the pre-heated oven at gas mark 5/375ºF/190ºC. Cook for 15-20 minutes until the cakes have risen. Place on a wire rack and allow to cool.

The mixture can also be cooked as a cake in a 7 inch tin for 45 minutes until the cake has risen.

Liver Puffs

These are very well received but are a bit of a faff to make so keep them for special occasions such as the end of course celebration at your dog club, or a doggie birthday party.

¼ lb liver
3 oz wholemeal macaroni
1 tablespoon flour
½ oz fat or 1 tablespoon vegetable oil
2 eggs
1 tablespoon chopped parsley
¼ milk

Cook the macaroni in boiling water until it is al dente, drain and allow to cool. In a small pan cook the liver gently in the fat or oil until it is quite firm. Remove from the pan and reserve. Make a sauce in the pan you used to cook the liver by adding the flour and milk and stirring until it is thick and lump free. Chop or mince the liver and macaroni and add to the sauce, also add the chopped parsley. Beat the eggs and add to the sauce mixture. Drop teaspoonfuls of the mixture into very hot fat in a deep fat fryer. They will puff up and be very light. Place on kitchen paper to cool. Store in an airtight container.

Fish

Dogs either love or hate fishy treats. Experiment to see if your dog is a fish lover. If he is, most of the above recipes can be adapted using any fish you like but oily fish is the strongest flavoured. Biscuits and puffs lend them selves best to fish, the bun recipe is not really suitable. Tinned fish such as sardines or mackerel can be used successfully but be warned; the smell of baking sardine biscuits is not to everyone's liking

Sardine Biscuits

Oil from a tin of sardines
1 or 2 sardines depending on size
1lb wholemeal flour

This is best made in a food processor. Place the wholemeal flour into the bowl of the processor, drain the oil from the tin of sardines onto the flour and blitz until you have a fine breadcrumb like mix. Mash the whole sardines and add to the flour and oil mix. Blitz for a few seconds so that the fish is evenly distributed throughout the mix. Add enough water a tablespoonful at a time to bring the mixture together into a dough. Turn out on to a floured board and roll out to about ¼ inch thick and cut into desired shapes. Close the kitchen door and open the windows. Place the biscuits on a baking tray and cook in the bottom of the oven at gas mark 3/325ºF/170ºC for 1 hour or until hard.

If your hands smell of sardine, rubbing them with a little lemon juice before washing should do the trick.

Anchovy Biscuits

These are one of the easiest and most popular fish treats.

1 tin anchovies
1 lb wholemeal flour
Water

Put the tin of anchovies into the bowl of the food processor with 2 tablespoons of water. Blitz until you have a runny paste. Add the flour and mix until you have dough. If necessary add a little extra water. Roll out and proceed as above.

Ice Cream

Dogs love ice cream especially on hot days. The ice cream we eat is a treat and an occasional small amount will do little harm. It is, however, very sugar heavy which is not good for our dogs teeth or blood sugar levels. Here are a couple of recipes for more dog-friendly ice creams that are fun to make and very popular as a fund raiser at doggie events. Both these ice creams have a high fat content so portions should be moderate. You can buy ready made ice cream cones or serve on a small digestive biscuit.

Vanilla Ice Cream 1

1½ tablespoons custard powder
¾ pint milk
¼ double cream
1 tablespoon malt extract
2 drops vanilla essence (optional)

Pour the double cream into a bowl, whip until it is thick but not stiff and place in the fridge to chill. In a pan mix 1½ tablespoons of custard powder with a little milk to make a smooth mixture. Add the malt extract and the vanilla essence and stir well. Put the pan on a low heat and gradually add the remaining milk, stirring all the time until the custard has thickened. It needs to be pouring consistency. Take off the heat, put into a bowl and allow to cool. It can be a good idea to put a piece of grease proof or butter paper on top of the custard to stop a skin forming. When the custard has cooled fold in the chilled cream and if you have an ice cream maker pour the mixture in to the bowl and allow to churn. Otherwise pour the mixture into a chilled bowl or polythene box and place in the freezer an hour or so until the mixture begins to set. When the mixture has reached this point take it out of the freezer and whisk thoroughly with a rotary whisk or electric beater to break up the ice crystals. When it is smooth return to the freezer where it need about 3 hours to become properly frozen. Take the ice cream out of the freezer about 30–45 minutes before serving.

Vanilla Ice Cream 2

400 gm can evaporated milk
1 tablespoon malt extract
1 oz corn flour
½ teaspoon vanilla essence

Chill the evaporated milk. While it is chilling mix the malt extract and the cornflour with the milk and cook for about 3 minutes until the mixture has thickened. Allow to cool. Whip the chilled evaporated milk until stiff and add to the cornflour mixture. Add the vanilla essence or any other flavouring you choose, beat well. Freeze.

Chocolate Ice Cream

This is not real chocolate ice cream it just looks like it.

Make a vanilla ice cream by your favourite method but mix two teaspoonsful of carob powder into the custard and proceed as normal. Carob contains lots of minerals but can be a little bitter so don't over do it, or add a little extra malt extract to taste.

Egg and Bacon Ice Cream

4 slices of fatty streaky bacon
2 eggs
¾ pint milk
¼ pint single cream

Gently grill the bacon on a piece of tin foil until it is nice and crispy. Remove the bacon and put to one side. Pour the fat from the bacon into a bowl and add the eggs, beat well. Now heat the milk and cream until nearly boiling and pour over the egg mixture, whisking well all the time. Place the bowl over a pan of not quite boiling water and continue whisking until the mixture has thickened. If the mixture looks as if it is curdling remove from the heat and continue whisking. It will go smooth again. Crumble the crispy bacon into the mixture and allow to cool. Pour the mixture into a bowl or plastic box in the freezer and whisk again after about 2 hours then return to the freezer for at least 3 hours. Alternatively you can use an ice cream maker.

Sweeties

Courgette Sweeties

½ lb courgettes (usually 2 smallish ones)
Scant ½ pint milk
2 cardamom pods
1 tablespoon vegetable oil
1 tablespoon malt extract

Wash and trim the courgettes. Grate coarsely and place in a wide, heavy pot. Add the milk and cardamom pods. Bring slowly to simmering point, turn the heat down slightly and cook, stirring from time to time to stop the mixture catching until the milk has almost evaporated. Remove the cardamon pods. Now add the oil and malt extract and stirring constantly cook until the mixture resembles mashed potatoes. Remove from the heat and stir for a further minute or so and then place the mixture in a greased tin and allow to cool. When the mixture is thoroughly cold cut into cubes.

Wholewheat Fudge

This is not fudge as we know it. This is doggie fudge. We use malt extract which is full of minerals to give a little sweetness and dogs love the smell.

2 oz butter
1 tablespoon vegetable oil
8 oz fine wholemeal flour
2 tablespoons malt extract

Boil some water, put it in a bowl and stand the jar of malt extract in it. This will make the extract easy to pour.

Meanwhile melt the butter and add the oil. If you prefer you can use oil only in which case it should be 3 tablespoons. Add the flour and cook for 5 minutes whilst stirring continuously to give a nice golden colour, now lower the heat and continue cooking for a further 10 minutes. Remove from heat. Now pour the malt extract on to the mixture and mix well. Spread the mixture on a greased tray making a 6 inch square about ½ inch thick. Allow to cool, then put in the fridge to chill and harden. Cut to desired size squares, small pieces are recommended.

Invalid Cookery

When your dog is under the weather or suffering from an illness the following recipes will stimulate the appetite and aid recovery. The following important points must be observed when catering for the invalid dog.

- Consult the vet as to the dog's diet and obey his instructions.
- Choose food which will supply the necessary nourishment and be suitable to the illness.
- Serve food which is easily digested because in sickness the digestive system is often impaired.
- Where the illness is serious food is often given in liquid form.
- When recovery is in progress see that food is light, easily digested and served only in small portions.
- As recovery proceeds, gradually increase the amount and variety of the food to stimulate the appetite.
- Avoid giving fatty or greasy food.
- Make sure that the food offered is absolutely fresh.
- Never leave uneaten food down. If your dog has no appetite remove the food and throw it away. Try again later with a fresh batch.
- Always have fresh water available.

Barley Water

This is helpful in cases of cystitis

1 oz pearl barley
1 pint water
1 teaspoon sugar

Wash the barley and put into a pan with the water. Bring very slowly to the boil and simmer for about 1 hour. Strain and allow to cool. This may be given on its own or diluted in the dogs drinking water.

Beef Tea

This is useful when solid food is being refused. It is relatively easy to open your dogs mouth and pour a little in, ensuring that some nourishment is given. When recovery is underway, mash a little brown rice or potato with some of this tea to make a cream like consistency.

½ lb lean steak. Cheap cuts such as shin or ox cheek are ideal.
½ pint water

Wipe the meat and remove any skin or fat. Chop finely or mince the meat and add to the water. Cover and allow to stand for about 30 mins. Put into a casserole dish, cover and put on the lowest shelf in the oven for 2 to 3 hours at gas mark 1/275ºF/135ºC. Strain and allow to cool. When cool remove any fat from the surface. Give small amounts from a spoon or water bottle. It is more palatable when luke warm.

If you are having difficulty in getting food into your dog a useful tip is to get some gelatine or agar agar and, following the instructions on the packet, make a jelly from the beef tea or chicken broth. It is then easy to pop a cube of jelly into a dogs mouth and it will melt as it goes down.

Chicken Essence

This is very restorative as it contains high levels of T cells which are an important part of the immune system.

½ lb chicken wings or a carcass of a roasted chicken
1 pint water

Wipe the chicken wings and chop into several pieces. Put into a pan with the water making sure the wings are covered. Bring slowly to the boil with the lid on the pan and simmer for about 2 hours or until the mixture cools to a jelly. Allow to cool and skim off any fat. Serve as above.

If you are using a chicken carcass, chop it into several pieces to allow the marrow to be released. You may find you need more water to cover the bones. Proceed as above.

Egg and Milk

1 egg
¼ pint Goats' milk

Beat the egg. Gently heat the goats milk and slowly add the beaten egg. Stir well until the mixture has thickened.

As you can see, this is really thickened milk or sloppy scrambled egg. When solid food is being taken you can give normal scrambled egg. Scrambled egg is easily digested and is very 'binding' so is helpful in digestive disorders.

Beef Tea Custard

This is given where extra nourishment is required.

1 egg
¼ pint beef tea

Beat the egg and add the beef tea. Pour into a small buttered basin and cover with greaseproof paper. Steam gently for 20 mins until set. Allow to cool.

Yogurt

Live yogurt should always be used. Both cows' and goats' milk yoghurts are readily available.

Yogurt is valuable in the treatment of upset stomachs, constipation, flatulence, and nervous fatigue.

Yogurt is easily digested and helps the intestines to synthesise vitamins K and B6. The friendly bacteria contained in yogurt combines with the good bacteria already in the gut providing protection from bad bacteria. Calcium is also better absorbed from yoghurt than from milk because of its acidity.

Yogurt should be given to your dog when a course of antibiotics is given in order to replace the intestinal flora killed off by the antibiotics. It should also form a regular part of your dog's diet. It may be given on its own or mixed with pulped meat or vegetables.

Bibliography

Prescription for Nutritional Healing, Balch and Balch

Complete Nutrition, Michael Sharon

Nutrients A-Z, Michael Sharon

Nutrient Requirements of Dogs and Cats, The National Accadamies Board on Agriculture and National Resources

All About The Greyhound, Anne Rollins

The Right Way To Keep Dogs, R C G Hancock

About Our Dogs, A Croxton Smith

Give Your Dog A Bone, Dr Ian Billinghirst

Border Collies, Iris Coombe

The Smallholders Encyclopedia

Dominance Fact or Fiction, Barry Eaton

Handbook of Applied Behaviour and Training, Steven Lindsay

All about The English Springer Spaniel, Olga M C Hampton

Poisionous Plants, www.takingthelead.co.uk

Essentials of Modern Cookery, Dora Seton

Farmhouse Recipes, W.I. collected Recipes 1954